Ginger & Turmeric
ZEN

By Roditch

Introduction

In the last five years, Ginger and Turmeric have become the superstars of health. I drink turmeric and ginger powder every day and they help me feel younger and healthier. I am not a doctor or a herbalist. 20 years ago when my daughter had the flu I was so worried about her I decided I had to do something that could help her get better and stop all the coughing, and discharging mucous from her lungs. At the time I was pretty busy teaching so every weekend I would come home and search for cures on the internet for the flu: I am still searching. Doctors like Dr. Axe https://draxe.com/ and Doctor Keith Scott-Mumby https://alternative-doctor.com/ and scientists like Mike Adams the Health Ranger https://www.naturalnews.com/ and Sayer Ji from www.greenmedinfo.com have made all the searching and research worthwhile.

When universities and renowned scientists are cited for doing substantial testing on ginger and turmeric, and then these findings are published by doctors, I feel confident about my health and my future health as should you. There is such a "good versus evil" side to this whole story which is getting more and more crazy every day. Researchers are now saying that ginger and turmeric are more effective at killing cancer than chemotherapy. What! Yes, that's right for as little as 10 dollars you can possibly treat your cancer better than going to the hospital and having chemotherapy (do all your research first). Ginger and turmeric are not the best anti-cancer treatments but the moment a doctor says you have cancer; at that moment, you have three choices: one is to go home and on the way buy some organic turmeric and ginger and take lots of it while you sort out what you do next. The second option is to stay and listen to all the expensive treatments your doctor will offer you to TRY and do it and the third option is to say hey doc I will try chemotherapy as long as you agree to me using a healthy routine in conjunction with the treatment like CBD oil, organic fruit, vegetable juicing, ginger and turmeric (curcumin form) and a host of other know proven cancer eradicators.

So, if you feel old and tired, you have aching joints, your libido is gone and you feel quite depressed, you are not alone, you have ginger and turmeric to help you get back on track. Many people who promote natural and healthy foods and supplements live in fear of large pharmacy companies cutting them down. Now is the best time to gather all the accurate information you can about cheap and natural healing substances: while you can.

Some of the many good points about turmeric and ginger are, they are easy to grow and you can cook delicious food with them. They will never be eradicated from our planet like Monsanto has eradicated original plant varieties and freedom of speech.

Whether you take them in your food, as a powder with water, or as pills, take them you should. They are food and a powerful herb at the same time. There are so many good herbs you can take for health and longevity; let's start with ginger and turmeric and make them part of your life, part of your daily routine, let's see after a month or two if you are feeling stronger, sexier, happier and healthier.

When writing about health I am aware of the need to convince everyone about "how good" herbs can be. In this small book, there will be many references to scientific studies and comments from Doctors and Scientists (in fact it is nearly all). I hope this will make you feel comfortable about using ginger and turmeric in your daily health routine. These two herbs are very popular worldwide and there has been tons of stuff written about them. This book is about how good these herbs are, as testified by science. There will be lots of advice on what to take them for, what doses and what side effects you have to know about. Even something like ginger beer that my father used to make has the potential for health: especially happiness health.

Back to trust for a minute. Even though this book is not huge and most of the information is coming from doctors and the NCBI I believe its true value is introducing you to something very special, something quite spiritual and something that is cheap but works incredibly well. Everyone these days need options for their health: all the possible options they can have to overcome disease. These options include traditional medicine, natural medicine, and innovative modern medicine. I do not believe doctors cover all these options apart from people like Dr. Axe. If they don't cover them all, then you need to. Yes, take responsibility for your preventive health care and cure.

The Blue Zones where a lot of people live to 100 years old are a great start to taking responsibility for your health: see the internet, blue zones. Entrusting your complete health care in a doctor is a mistake as is entrusting your soul to a preacher and your economy to a politician. You must take 'control'. Start your personal 'wonderful life' notebook and add little treasures every day, and as you add them, do them, after 30 days you will feel better in every way.

Alcohol is quite bad for you but when made 'organically and in moderation' it is good for you. There are many studies that say we all should drink a glass of wine every day (especially homemade wine) some dark chocolate and two cups of organic coffee.

I don't drink much. I have one glass of beer every week. In my heart of hearts, I am a monk. I want a peaceful spiritual communion with everything my soul can know and be. I don't like fun, "think of all the good times I've been wasting having good times" The Rolling Stones. I would rather do something inspiring than get drunk or eat a giant steak. Life is full of promise and potential: this is completely halted in the pursuit of fun. As easy as it seems to take care of our health: it's nearly impossible for most of us. Whatever program we have in our heads telling us to drink and stuff ourselves with food, usually comes from the past, way back when. Once you accept that you eat too much junk food, drink too much, chase after women and money too much, watch too much TV, are scared of nearly everything and can't talk about how you really feel to anyone then it's time to take ginger and turmeric every day and let them save you. You will feel more balanced in every part of your life. Once you have read this book, you can learn heaps more if you need to on the internet: depending on what your illness is. This is the start.

Eat to live
or live to eat.

   This is a serious question we must all ask ourselves: especially when we really do need to change our diet to a much healthier one. In our mundane lives, eating comes first as "a pleasure" before shopping, religion, and sex. I have always been pretty moderate about 'fun' all my life. I would rarely feel passionate about drinking, eating, religion or sex. My joy comes from studying herbs, reading about spiritual subjects, playing music and having loving and peaceful relationships.

   When my friends get excited about food and plan dinner at a restaurant and buy an expensive bottle of wine, my mind wanders to a poem or some inspiring idea. Crayfish, oysters, steak, red wine, cake, and coffee all blend into 'normal'. I am not looking for rewards for working hard: I don't enjoy three hours of eating and talking as a means to happiness. I prefer a quiet time thinking about life and the state of the world. So it's pretty easy for me to eat healthy food because I get excited about eating food I know is good for me.

   My father was interested in healthy food and nutrition which was a good starting point. He was before the lentil revolution so the food he actually eat every day was normal food. He liked crayfish, curried sausages, rollmops, and Shepherd's Pie. When I was 18 everything started changing. All the Italian, Greek, and Turkish migrants started opening restaurants and their national dishes included lots of healthy food that I had never heard of like garlic, yogurt, fava beans, and parsley: mainly vegetarian fare.

Now there are so many options when it comes to eating mainstream food that originates from other countries: we are so lucky. Yet, we are all getting sicker, especially cancer and heart disease, why is this? The answer is we are all in a hurry. This means not only are we suffering from stress which is very unhealthy we also don't have the time or the money to take care of ourselves. Maybe if doctors kept nagging us to change our diet and lifestyle to one full of organic fruit and vegetables, regular exercise and take herbs for health not pharmaceuticals we could change our ways easier: but they don't. On the topic of changing our ways and eating to live instead of living to eat we are on our own pretty much; well that was before the internet. Now even if we can't get help locally to improve our wellbeing it is available on the internet with people like Dr. Axe.

Instead of stressing out, (even more) about changing our diets and menus we can start just by listening and reading and building up a body of knowledge first, which will help us take the next step: creating new food and medicine routines that will make us much healthier and stronger.

Junk food given to children on their birthdays is a huge mistake because you are telling them that it is special and that whenever you can get junk food in the future you will be happy because it is so wonderful. And even when you are all grown up and celebrate special times like birthdays you feel like you must eat junky food or it isn't any fun: this is wrong thinking.

What has this got to do with ginger and turmeric? Ginger and turmeric are part of a new way of thinking and acting. They need you to change your habits and inner emotional desires for "junk fun" so that you will actually see them every day in your food and drinks. This will mean reprogramming your mind—which can be done in 30 days. We are all, including me, victims of the past. So many of our actions stem from past memories and situations (locked away in our subconscious). A good example is men wanting their new wives to cook just like their mother did. Another good example is of the chain smoker who can't stop smoking but their health is going down the toilet fast. They know it's killing them but can't stop. I think the reason they can't stop is because when they first started to smoke it made them feel all grown up: which means handsome, strong, and sexy. Now, 40 years later they think, their subconscious thinks, that if they give up they will lose all those wonderful attributes and benefits. One more example is of a man in his 60's who had big dreams and no money. For years he dreamt about buying a big truck and building a shed for it. When his father died he got a lot of money from his inheritance. He spent it all on a truck and a shed in the first two weeks. But, there was a problem: he didn't need a truck or a shed anymore. He was too old to drive one. The power of thought, dreams, desires, sit, unchallenged in our subconscious until we become superheroes and go into battle with it: reprogram outdated thoughts and behavior and do a big RESET. One way of doing this is taking action. No matter how small: take the steps. The first step will lead to another step then another and soon you will have traveled further than you ever could have dreamed.

It seems bizarre to think a big RESET can be one small step but it's true and never forget it; during those times you want to give up. There will be moments when your mind is telling you (from your subconscious, which doesn't want to change) you can't do it, you have no money, this is bollocks, listen to your doctor, how you can you achieve such a large goal with so little time. Again, the answer is always action: to overcome your lying and unhelpful mind and the beauty is: these actions can be small and still end up being big and breaking the power of your subconscious mind. Small is Big.

I am struggling every day with my subconscious. I have many things that can be improved in my life, especially around self-confidence and love. The one big reason we all struggle is because it is sub: under our conscious (our awareness) so we can't see our enemy, or know what it's up to and where it is. Sometimes other people (ones who love us) give advice we should listen to. Psychologists are trained to work out these issues and when life just seems too crazy you get glimpses of what is not working and something needs changing: you need to take action as soon as you realize before you go back to being ignorant.

I love ginger and Turmeric: without them, I would not have the energy and courage to go on and do more battles with my past and the future.

Ginger

Ginger is both delicious and healthy. It has been used all around the world for centuries. The health benefits of ginger are largely due to its antioxidants, anti-inflammatory properties, and content of therapeutic compounds like gingerol. You can take it fresh, as powder, in your food and tea, or in capsule form. Ginger, also known as Zingiber officinale, is a flowering plant that is closely related to turmeric and cardamom.

My family grows organic ginger. We wash it, dry it and I then make it into powder. Every day I put two teaspoons of the powder in my mouth and let it slowly dissolve and then I swallow it. It is pretty spicy but I don't mind because I like to eat a lot of fresh chilies every day too. Sometimes I stop doing this routine and when I do my energy levels go down, my libido definitely goes down and I am more likely to catch the flu from my young students. I have definitely invited ginger into my life and I am so grateful for its existence. My wife and I make ginger beer which is to die for: so refreshing and yummy—and easy to make. https://www.youtube.com/watch?v=8dWbTEfg-tk I also, sometimes, have a cup of ginger tea. There are many stir fries and soups we can put ginger in too.

I love to eat candied ginger, whenever I can get it, and I often make ginger syrup to keep away the flu and give it to my friends (boil some fresh ginger, in filtered water and brown sugar, and put it into a jar).

Without Ginger life would be horrible. I would get old so much quicker, I would always walk around complaining of aches and pains, definitely have low levels of testosterone in my body, and food would taste awful. Ginger is part of my SIMPLE philosophy which is how I want to live my life these days. I have discovered simple is not easy, but it is best way to do things. Simple love, simple health, simple religion, and simple fun. Ginger fits into most of these categories very well. Ginger will definitely improve your love life. Ginger improves your health. Ginger is one of God's (God is everything above me) herbs: given with love. Ginger products are always delicious and zesty, and so enjoyable to eat.

NCBI

National Center for Biotechnology Information

The **National Center for Biotechnology Information** (NCBI)
is part of the United States National Library of Medicine
(NLM), a branch of the National Institutes of Health (NIH).
https://www.ncbi.nlm.nih.gov/home/about/
https://en.wikipedia.org/wiki/National_Center_for_Biotec
hnology_Information

This small book continually refers to studies done by the
NCBI so you can have scientific proof of the veracity of
natural cures. These are good times for people who are
cynics, disbelievers, and "behind the times". Now you have
the reassurance you need to "bump up against" your
doctor when choosing treatments (you can print these out
and show them to him or her). Now you can manage a
large part of your own treatment independently of doctors
and hospitals if you are prepared to put in the time
studying what protocols will work for you and then putting
them into action. There are a growing number of people
who are choosing both: some treatment by a doctor and
some treatment using natural remedies and diets. Now
CBD oil is going mainstream it has just got a lot easier to
cure diseases yourself. CBD Oil used in conjunction with
other therapies will probably be what doctors use in the
next five years.

I have personally seen doctors fail, again and again, to
cure people of major disease, resulting in the premature
death of their patients. It is criminal that people are
suffering financially, physically and emotionally because
doctors are controlling the health agenda along with

pharmaceutical companies. I believe we all should use the very best treatments available NOW to prevent and cure major diseases like Cancer and Heart attacks. Doctors do not have the best cures: in fact, they make more money if you stay sick which is a huge conflict of interest.

I suggest, you do your homework and build a small library of REAL (start with NCBI) cures and health promoting herbs and supplements to use as the foundations of your health, and find a natural doctor.

The obvious ones to start with are moderate daily exercise, pure water, and fresh air. Some sun on your skin as often as possible: maybe a sunbath around 10 in the morning. Eat a diet full of good oils like avocado, olive, and coconut.

Lots of organic fruit and vegetables. Nuts and seeds from all around the world. Probiotics and prebiotics like kefir, yogurt, kimchi, garlic, onion, black sesame seed hulls and flaxseed hulls. Some good quality wine, dark chocolate, and organic coffee. Daily meditation and yoga are a pretty essential part of your routine too and happiness, fun, family, friends, and community.

A spiritual practice like Christianity, Hinduism, do your own thing ism or Buddhism. Be creative, paint, write a book, sing, and dance. Use more natural cosmetics and toiletries. Open your mind to everything. Try to avoid party politics and function more as a unifier than disunifier (we are all one big family). Ginger and Turmeric are right up there as part of your health foundation because they are so cheap and easy to incorporate into your daily routine; they are very close to the top of your list of things to do.

Helps Treat Nausea

Ginger is a natural remedy for seasickness and morning sickness.
https://www.ncbi.nlm.nih.gov/pmc/articles/PMC3995184/
It is also effective in reducing nausea with patients receiving chemotherapy.
https://www.ncbi.nlm.nih.gov/pubmed/21818642/

"The most effective natural thing is ginger root," said Dr. Michelle Collins, a certified nurse-midwife and director of the nurse-midwifery program at Vanderbilt University School of Nursing in Nashville, Tenn. Ginger ale and ginger snaps, however, probably won't help because they're not made with enough real ginger. Instead, drink ginger root boiled in water, or look for ginger root tea, ginger beer (it's nonalcoholic), lozenges, gum or capsules.

   The rhizome of *Zingiber officinale*, commonly known as ginger, has been used as a nausea remedy in various traditional systems of medicine for more than 2,000 years. Many preclinical and clinical studies have shown ginger to possess nausea-reducing effects against different stimuli.
   In 2000, researchers at the School of Postgraduate Medicine and Health Sciences in the U.K. performed a systematic review of the evidence from randomized controlled trials for or against the efficacy of ginger for nausea and vomiting. One study was found for each of the following conditions: seasickness, morning sickness and chemotherapy-induced nausea. The studies collectively favored ginger over placebo.

To get rid of nausea and take advantage of the medicinal ginger health benefits, drink ginger tea throughout the day. To make your own ginger tea, cut ginger root into slices and place them into a pot of boiling water for 10 minutes. Then strain the ginger, and you're ready to drink. You can also find ginger tea at most grocery stores. In addition, you can use ginger essential oil if you prefer that route.

(Dr. Axe, Christine Ruggeri, February 11, 2016)

Fungal Infections

Fungal infections cause a wide variety of conditions, from yeast infections to jock itch and athlete's foot. Fortunately, ginger helps kill off disease-causing fungi due to its powerful anti-fungal properties. Ginger extract is effective against two types of yeast that commonly cause fungal infections in the mouth.

https://www.ncbi.nlm.nih.gov/pubmed/27127591

Ginger is one of the most effective of all plants at killing fungus.

An article about ginger and garlic killing fungus on fish.

https://www.researchgate.net/publication/279924216_ANTI-FUNGAL_PROPERTIES_OF_GINGER_ZINGIBER_OFFICINALE_AND_GARLIC_ALLIUM_SATIVUM_ON_SMOKED_CAT_FISH_MYCOFLORA

(The American Journal of applied sciences)
Our study focused on the effect of ginger extract on the oral species of Candida (Albicans) and showed the significant anticandidal effect of the extract.

https://www.thescipub.com/pdf/10.3844/ajassp.2009.1067.1069

Eases Menstrual Pains

Two studies show how effective Ginger is in relieving the pain, headaches, and cramps associated with menstruation. That it is equal to or better than most pain killers. https://www.ncbi.nlm.nih.gov/pubmed/19216660 and
https://www.ncbi.nlm.nih.gov/pmc/articles/PMC3518208/

Research suggests that compounds found in ginger may help to protect against the increases in inflammation, by inhibiting the body's production of prostaglandins (a class of pro-inflammatory chemicals involved in triggering the muscle contractions that help the uterus shed its lining). Because the onset of menstrual cramps appears to be linked to excessive production of prostaglandins, it's thought that consuming ginger in dietary supplement or tea form can help reduce menstrual pain.

Studies published in recent years suggest that ginger may be helpful for the relief of dysmenorrhea (the medical term for pain before or during menstruation).
A report published in *Pain Medicine* in 2015, for instance, scientists looked at previously published trials testing the effects on ginger in women with dysmenorrhea not caused by pelvic conditions such as endometriosis. In their analysis, the report's authors found that was more effective than a placebo in relieving pain.

Another **report**, published in 2016, examined previously published studies on the use of ginger for dysmenorrhea.

Ginger was found to be more effective than a placebo in reducing pain severity. Of the two studies comparing ginger to a nonsteroidal anti-inflammatory drug (NSAID), ginger was found to be as effective at reducing pain.

In addition, there's some evidence that ginger may help control heavy menstrual bleeding. In a clinical trial published in *Phytotherapy Research* in 2015, for instance, 92 women with heavy menstrual bleeding were treated with either ginger or a placebo for three menstrual periods. At the end of the study, researchers found that levels of menstrual blood loss dramatically declined among study participants who received ginger.

(Cathy Wong, Very Well Health, October 15, 2018)
https://www.verywellhealth.com/ginger-for-menstrual-cramps-90072

Stomach Ulcers

Stomach ulcers are painful sores that cause symptoms like indigestion, fatigue, heartburn and stomach pain. Several studies have found that ginger could help prevent the formation of stomach ulcers.
https://www.ncbi.nlm.nih.gov/pmc/articles/PMC3763798/

"The rhizomes of Zingiber officinale Roscoe (Zingiberaceae), commonly known as ginger is an important kitchen spice and also possess myriad health benefits. The rhizomes have been used since antiquity in the various traditional systems of medicine to treat arthritis, rheumatism, sprains, muscular aches, pains, sore throats, cramps, hypertension, dementia, fever, infectious diseases, catarrh, nervous diseases, gingivitis, toothache, asthma, stroke, and diabetes. Ginger is also used as a home remedy and is of immense value in treating various gastric ailments like constipation, dyspepsia, belching, bloating, gastritis, epigastric discomfort, gastric ulcerations, indigestion, nausea and vomiting, and scientific studies have validated the ethnomedicinal uses. Ginger is also shown to be effective in preventing gastric ulcers induced by nonsteroidal anti-inflammatory drugs [NSAIDs like indomethacin, aspirin], reserpine, ethanol, stress (hypothermic and swimming), acetic acid and Helicobacter pylori-induced gastric ulcerations in laboratory animals."
(NCBI, 2013)

https://www.ncbi.nlm.nih.gov/pubmed/23612703

Ginger Inhibits Cancer Growth

One of the most impressive benefits of ginger is its anti-cancer properties, thanks to the presence of a powerful compound called 6-gingerol. That it may be effective in blocking cancer cell growth and development for ovarian, pancreatic and prostate cancer shown by these studies.

https://www.ncbi.nlm.nih.gov/pmc/articles/PMC2241638/
https://www.ncbi.nlm.nih.gov/pmc/articles/PMC2687755/
https://www.ncbi.nlm.nih.gov/pubmed/21849094

Some of the most studied actions of ginger are its analgesic and anti-inflammatory effects through the inhibition of NF-kB, COX-2, and 5-LOX (the major pathways and switches of inflammation mentioned previously). Ginger also has been shown to protect against cancers and to demonstrate a chemoprotective effect, meaning it protects the body from the side effects of chemotherapy. Some characteristics of ginger's actions include the following: [2]

Induction of apoptosis (programmed cell death) of cancer cells
Inhibits IkBa kinase activation (upregulates apoptosis)
Upregulation of BAX (a proapoptosis gene)
Downregulation of Bcl-2 proteins (cancer associated)

Downregulation of prosurvival genes (anti-apoptotic) Bcl-xl, Mcl-1, and Survivin

Downregulation of cell-cycle-regulating proteins, including cyclin D1 and cyclin-dependent kinase 4 (CDK4) (cancer associated)

Increased expression of CDK inhibitor, p21 (anticancer associated)

Inhibition of c-Myc, hTERT (cancer associated)

Abolishes RANKL-induced NF-kB activation

Inhibits osteoclastogenesis (type of bone cell that breaks down bone tissue to remodel and repair)

Suppresses human breast-cancer-induced bone loss

If you or a loved one has been stricken with cancer, then you probably know the importance of all of these functions. Thus, it's easy to see that ginger can play an important role in regulating not only inflammation but also various signals that affect cancer cells.

Ginger and its constituents have been shown to inhibit the following cancers:

Breast cancer, Colon and rectal cancer, Leukemia, Liver cancer, Lung cancer, Melanoma, Pancreatic cancer, Prostate cancer, Skin cancer and Stomach cancer.

To demonstrate just how important ginger can be to helping eliminate cancers, let's look at one example: ovarian cancer.

In ovarian cancer, there are usually some indicators of the inflammation, such as vascular endothelial growth factor (VEGF), interleukin-8, and prostaglandin E2 (PEG2). Ginger extracts have been shown to greatly decrease these inflammatory markers in ovarian cancer patients. [4] Thus not only can it be taken as a tea or food to help warm someone who may feel cold or have nausea (especially those being treated with chemotherapy), but ginger also has a beneficial effect for those with serious health conditions like ovarian cancer.

Another interesting aspect of ginger is its hypoglycemic effect against enzymes linked to type 2 diabetes. Anyone who has diabetes or even mild insulin resistance can enjoy this added benefit of ginger; it is not harmful to those who are taking diabetes medication. Instead, it may improve overall glucose control. In addition, keeping blood glucose in the lower/normal range is optimal for those with cancer, even if they do not have diabetes.

To sum up, ginger is a strong antioxidant that can help with metabolic syndrome, diabetes, cardiovascular disease, dementia, and inflammatory conditions such as arthritis, osteoporosis, and even cancers. Thus, in addition to taking Bosmeric-SR, one should try to include organic ginger in the diet as much as possible. Try adding it to foods like salsa, smoothies, or stir-fry. Ginger is a staple in most Thai and Indian curries and sauces, which are both fun and easy to make at home to liven up the flavors of any meal. You can also cut off half an inch of organic ginger root and blend it in a juicer along with other veggies and fruits to give your juice a kick of spiciness. For those with weak digestion, see *Ginger Elixir Recipe* to jump-start your digestive system before meals.

(Cancer Tutour, 2019)
https://www.cancertutor.com/ginger-fighting-cancer/

Prostate Cancer

Ginger rhizome is extensively used in the form of a fresh paste or dried powder to flavor food and beverages in places such as India and China[14]. The present study reports a novel finding that oral consumption of the extract of whole ginger, a commonly consumed vegetable worldwide, significantly inhibits prostate tumor progression in both *in vitro* and *in vivo* mice models. The anticancer effect of GE was coupled with its significant antiproliferative, cell-cycle inhibitory and pro-apoptotic activity in cell culture as well as in prostate tumor xenograft models.

https://www.ncbi.nlm.nih.gov/pmc/articles/PMC3426621/

This is very encouraging "proof" that ginger is well worth taking to not only prevent cancer but cure it as well.

Breast Cancer

Study finds Ginger is powerful in treating breast cancer
PLOS has many studies in their library about Ginger
https://www.plos.org/search?q=ginger

A new study published in PLoS (Public Library of Science www.plos.org) reveals that ginger contains a pungent compound, known as 6-shogaol which could be up to 10,000 times more effective than conventional chemotherapy in targeting the root cause of breast cancer malignancy: namely, the breast cancer stem cells.

Cancer stem cells are at the root of a wide range of cancers, not just breast cancer, and are sometimes referred to as "mother cells" because they are responsible for producing all the different "daughter" cell types that make up the tumor colony. While cancer stem cells only constitute between .2 and 1% of the cells within any given tumor, they have the seeming "immortal" ability to self-renew, are capable of continuous differentiation, are resistant to conventional chemotherapeutic agents, and are tumorigenic, i.e. are capable of "splitting off" to create new tumor colonies. Clearly, the cancer stem cells within a tumor must be destroyed if cancer treatment is to effect a lasting cure.

The new study titled, "6-Shogaol Inhibits Breast Cancer Cells and Stem Cell-Like Spheroids by Modulation of Notch Signaling Pathway and Induction of Autophagic Cell Death, (https://journals.plos.org/plosone/article?id=10.1371/journal.pone.0137614) " identified powerful anti-cancer stem cell activity in 6-shogaol, a compound of ginger produced when the root is either dried or cooked. The study also found that the cancer-destroying effects occurred at concentrations that were non-toxic to non-cancerous cells – a crucial difference from conventional cancer treatments that do not exhibit this kind of selective cytotoxicity.

The researchers identified a variety of ways by which 6-shagoal targets breast cancer:

It reduces the expression of CD44/CD24 cancer stem cell surface markers in breast cancer spheroids (3-dimensional cultures of cells modeling stem cell like cancer)

It significantly affects the cell cycle, resulting in increased cancer cell death

It induces programmed cell death primarily through the induction of autophagy, with apoptosis a secondary inducer, It inhibits breast cancer spheroid formation by altering Notch signaling pathway through γ-secretase inhibition.It exhibits cytotoxicity (cell killing properties) against monolayer (1-dimensional cancer model) and spheroid cells (3-dimensional cancer model)

It was in evaluating the last mode of 6-shagoal's chemotherapeutic activity and comparing it to the activity of the conventional chemotherapeutic agent taxol that the researchers discovered an astounding difference. Whereas taxol exhibited clear cytotoxicity in the one-dimensional (flat) monolayer experimental model, it had virtually no effect on the spheroid model, which is a more "real world" model reflecting the 3-dimensionality of tumors and their stem cell sub-populations.

This is a highly significant finding, as it affirms a common theme in cancer research that acknowledges the primary role of cancer stem cells: while conventional techniques like surgery, radiation, and chemotherapy are effective at reducing a tumor's size, sometimes to the point where it is "poisoned" out of the body, the appearance of "beating cancer" often comes at a steep price. Ultimately, the cancer stem cell population may regrow the tumors, which now exhibit an increased vengeance.

In their concluding remarks, the authors point out a hugely important distinction between natural anti-cancer agents and conventional ones that have only been introduced in the past half-century or so. Unlike modern synthetically-produced and patented chemicals, ginger, curcumin, green tea, and hundreds of other compounds naturally found in the human diet, have been "time-tested" as acceptable to the human body in the largest and longest running "clinical trials" known: the tens of thousands of years of direct human experience, spanning thousands of different cultures from around the world, that constitute human prehistory.

(PLOS.org)

Regulating Blood Sugar

High blood sugar can cause many negative symptoms, from frequent urination to headaches and increased thirst Research shows that ginger helps promote normal blood sugar.

https://www.ncbi.nlm.nih.gov/pmc/articles/PMC4277626/

   A study published in the August 2012 edition of the natural product journal Planta Medica suggested that ginger may improve long-term blood sugar control for people with **type 2 diabetes.**
   Researchers from the University of Sydney, Australia, found that extracts from Buderim Ginger (Australian grown ginger) rich in gingerols - the major active component of the ginger rhizome - can increase uptake of glucose into muscle cells without using insulin, and may, therefore, assist in the management of high blood sugar levels.
   In the December 2009 issue of the European Journal of Pharmacology, researchers reported that two different ginger extracts, spissum and an oily extract, interact with serotonin receptors to reveres their effect on insulin secretion. Treatment with the extracts led to a 35 percent drop in blood glucose levels and a 10 percent increase in plasma insulin levels.
   A study published in the August 2010 edition of Molecular Vision revealed that a small daily dose of ginger helped delay the onset and progression of cataracts - one of the sight-related complications of long-term diabetes -

in diabetic rats.

It's also worth noting that ginger has a very low **glycemic index (GI).** Low GI foods break down slowly to form glucose and therefore do not trigger a spike in blood sugar levels as high GI foods do.

Ginger has been used as an herbal therapy in Chinese, Indian, and Arabic medicine for centuries to aid digestion, combat the common cold and relieve pain. Its powerful anti-inflammatory substances, gingerols, make it an effective pain reliever and it is commonly used to reduce pain and swelling in patients with arthritis and those suffering from other inflammation and muscle complaints. In fact, ginger is said to be just as effective as nonsteroidal anti-inflammatory drugs, but without the gastro-intestinal side effects.

Relieves Joint
and Muscle Pain

Because of its ability to reduce inflammation, adding ginger into your diet could help treat both muscle pain and arthritis-related joint pain. There are many studies that show how well Ginger works in reducing inflammation and pain in joints and muscles.
https://www.ncbi.nlm.nih.gov/pubmed/20418184

and this one on knee pain.
https://www.ncbi.nlm.nih.gov/pubmed/11710709

Besides being a tasty spice often used to enhance holiday treats, ginger can soothe upset stomachs and diminish nausea, and studies show it may help pain and inflammation, too.

In fact, a University of Miami study concluded that ginger extract could one day be a substitute to nonsteroidal anti-inflammatory drugs (NSAIDs). The study compared the effects of a highly concentrated ginger extract to placebo in 247 patients with osteoarthritis (OA) of the knee. The ginger reduced pain and stiffness in knee joints by 40 percent over the placebo.

"Research shows that ginger affects certain inflammatory processes at a cellular level," says the study's lead author, Roy Altman, MD, now at the University of California, Los Angeles. What makes ginger so helpful? "Ginger has anti-inflammatory, anti-ulcer and antioxidant activities, as well as a small amount of analgesic property," says Roberta Lee, MD, vice chair of the Department of Integrative Medicine at Beth Israel Medical Center in New York City.

Choosing the most effective form of ginger may be the biggest challenge to reaping its rewards. Ginger comes in capsules, tinctures, teas, powders, oils, and foods made from the dried or fresh root of the ginger plant. While many forms of ginger boast health benefits, Dr. Lee says capsules provide better benefits than other forms. She advises people to look for brands that use "super-critical extraction," because it results in the purest ginger and will provide the greatest effect. She also suggests taking ginger capsules with food. Why? Although small amounts of ginger can help settle a sour stomach, concentrated doses can actually cause stomach upset.

Although they smell wonderful, foods like gingerbread, gingersnaps and ginger tea may not contain enough ginger to have an effect, says Dr. Altman. The capsule taken twice daily by patients in Dr. Altman's study contained 255 milligrams (mg) of ginger, the equivalent of nearly a bushel of your grocer's ginger.

Try a 100- to 200-mg ginger capsule each day for four to six weeks to see if you feel an effect. Steer clear of ginger if you're taking a blood-thinning medication, like warfarin (*Coumadin*), as ginger may reverse the effects of these types of drugs.

If you prefer the tangy zip of fresh ginger, here's some good news. Researchers at the University of Georgia in Athens and Georgia State College & University in Milledgeville reported in the *Journal of Pain* that a few tablespoons of grated ginger can help ease muscle pain caused by exercise. You can add a few tablespoons to your diet by grating ginger over a salad or into a stir fry.

Or you could grate one to two teaspoons and simmer it in a pot with hot water for five minutes to make a soothing tea. (Arthritis Today Magazine, 2019)

Ginger lowers Cholesterol Levels

One of the biggest benefits of ginger is its ability to naturally lower cholesterol levels and triglycerides to reduce your risk of heart problems.
Here is a study that shows that Ginger can reduce bad LDL cholesterol.

https://www.ncbi.nlm.nih.gov/pubmed/18813412

and another study that shows Ginger is as effective at lowering cholesterol as top cholesterol medication.

https://www.ncbi.nlm.nih.gov/pubmed/23901210

The human heart beats around 70 times a minute, non-stop for 80 years give or take, pumping more than 10 million litres of blood around your body every year. Without a break, it continues its steady, faithful beat. Sadly, many of us take our hearts for granted. Heart disease accounts for 1 in 4 deaths in the United States and around 600,000 people die of heart disease in the U.S. every year. Heart disease is the leading cause of death for both men and women.

Research shows that ginger may play a role in maintaining a healthy heart. Used in traditional Chinese, Indonesian and Ayurvedic medicine, ginger has been used for centuries to treat a variety of cardiovascular conditions. In theory, ginger helps reduce your risk of heart attack and stroke. But how does ginger do this?

Studies have shown that ginger contains anti-inflammatory properties that work much like the more common non-steroidal anti-inflammatory drugs, often referred to as NSAIDs. 1 Specifically, ginger inhibits the action of several of the genes involved in the inflammation process. Ginger helps to reduce inflammation by actually blocking the very genes needed to create inflammation in the first place.

In a placebo-controlled animal study, researchers gave both a low dose (50 mg/kg) and a high dose (500 mg/kg) of ginger extract to rats for four weeks. 2 Researchers found that rats given the higher dosage of ginger extract orally exhibited a statistically significant reduction in blood-clotting factors and cholesterol levels, as compared to the placebo group. They also had a reduction in inflammation markers. Researchers concluded that ginger may be useful as a cholesterol-lowering, anti-inflammatory blood thinner.

The University of Maryland Medical Center cites a number of studies that suggest ginger may lower cholesterol and prevent blood from clotting. This blood-thinning or anti-coagulant effect is important for people with heart disease: if blood is thinner and free-flowing, it is much less likely to become clogged and lead to a heart attack or stroke. Studies at Cornell University point specifically to the 'gingerols' in ginger as being responsible for helping to prevent abnormal blood coagulation.

Buckle up for the science part about cholesterol: a type of fat, cholesterol is found in all cells in the body (it forms part of their outer layer) and is

transported around the body, in the blood, attached to a protein. This combination of fat and protein is called a lipoprotein. Lipoproteins can be high density (HDL) or low density (LDL). Although we often hear how cholesterol is bad for us (and too much of the wrong type is), some cholesterol is actually essential for good health.

HDL cholesterol is mostly made up of protein and a small amount of fat. It helps to protect against heart disease by transporting fats away from the arteries and is often referred to as 'good' cholesterol. LDL cholesterol is made up of mostly fat and a small amount of protein. It can cause cholesterol levels to build up in the arteries, increasing the risk of heart disease and is often referred to as 'bad' cholesterol. Some studies go further and suggest that this is just half the story: it's not just about the good and the bad, but also other factors such as oxidative stress and inflammation.

What is key, is balance: high levels of HDL and low levels of LDL, and many studies show that ginger reduces blood cholesterol levels (probably by reducing inflammation and oxidative stress) and also by improving liver function. Ginger may also help lower blood pressure, another indicator of heart disease.

https://gingerpeople.com/news/love-ginger-love-your-heart/

Grzanna, R et al. "Ginger – an herbal medicinal product with broad anti- inflammatory actions." J Med Food. 2005 Summer;8(2):125-32.

Thomson, M et al. "The use of ginger (Zingiber officinale Rosc.) as a potential anti-inflammatory and antithrombotic agent." Prostaglandins Leukot Essent Fatty Acids. 2002 Dec;67(6):475-8.

Verma, SK et al. "Antioxidant property of ginger in patients with coronary artery disease." South Asian J Prev Cardiology. 2004;8

Ginger Improves Brain Function

Neurodegenerative conditions like Alzheimer's disease and Parkinson's have been linked to oxidative stress and chronic inflammation in the brain. With its wealth of antioxidants and potent anti-inflammatory properties, ginger is believed to play an important role in the health of your brain. Several animal studies have found that ginger extract could protect against brain aging and cognitive decline. (used in conjunction with turmeric and fish oil these results would be much greater)

Alzheimers -
https://www.ncbi.nlm.nih.gov/pubmed/23374025 and
https://www.ncbi.nlm.nih.gov/pubmed/20952170

also this study showing Ginger improves brain function in women.
https://www.ncbi.nlm.nih.gov/pmc/articles/PMC3253463/

Ginger Blocks Bacterial Infections

In addition to its antifungal properties, ginger boasts the ability to fight off bacterial infections as well. Pathogenic bacteria are common culprits behind conditions like urinary tract infections, pneumonia and bronchitis. This study shows how Ginger can inhibit bacteria that causes gum disease.
https://www.ncbi.nlm.nih.gov/pubmed/18814211 and this study how effective Ginger is with many strains of bacteria.
https://www.ncbi.nlm.nih.gov/pmc/articles/PMC3609356/

Ginger can be used as an antibiotic agent because of its ability to treat infections in the body. Say, for example, there are types of respiratory problems and all of them are caused by infection from bacteria and viruses, which may trigger secretion of mucus, phlegm and an increased risk of inflammation. Ginger can soothe and treat these problems. In some developing countries, many children die because of diarrhea. Diarrhea itself is not the cause of death, but the toxins that may spread throughout the body as a result of diarrhea are the culprits. Zingerone, an active compound found in ginger, can gather the toxins so they can't affect the stomach. It can prevent bacterial diarrhea. However, children who are less than 2 years old shouldn't take ginger because of some side effects. Before giving any herbal medicine to children, consult with your doctor first. (visihow, 2019)
https://visihow.com/Use_Ginger_As_Antiseptic_or_Antibacterial_Agent

Ginger Eases Inflammation

Although inflammation can be a normal, healthy immune response to injury and infection, chronic inflammation is believed to be a major contributor to conditions like heart disease, obesity, diabetes and cancer.

https://www.ncbi.nlm.nih.gov/pmc/articles/PMC3492709/ and
https://www.ncbi.nlm.nih.gov/pmc/articles/PMC3665023/ and
https://www.ncbi.nlm.nih.gov/pmc/articles/PMC3665023/

Ginger is mostly famous for its ability to combat nausea and motion sickness, as well as ease the symptoms of many gastrointestinal disorders. However, ginger can also help reduce inflammation as a result of its high levels of gingerols. For that reason, ginger should be considered as an all-natural remedy for treating a wide variety of inflammatory ailments, from migraines and headaches, to sore muscles, arthritic joints, and even menstrual cramps.

Inflammation is a general term that refers to when part of your body becomes swollen and painful. Inflammation is usually characterized by redness on the affected area, and can be triggered by many things, including overexertion, immune response to pathogens, injuries, and the effects of chemicals or radiation. One type of inflammation that can be treated with ginger is muscle soreness.

Ginger is most effective in treating inflammation caused by oxidative stress - an imbalance between the production of free radicals and the body's antioxidant defenses, which has been linked to conditions such as atherosclerosis, hypertension, diabetes mellitus, cancer, and ischemic diseases.

As mentioned previously, ginger properties include anti-inflammatory actions that stem from a group of compounds called gingerols, which work by inhibiting the prostaglandin-biosynthesizing enzyme, known as PH synthetase or cyclooxygenase (COX). Depending on which of the many medicinal uses of ginger is preferred, the gingerols break down into two other types of compounds. When ginger is cooked, the gingerols are transformed into become shogaols, while in dried ginger zingerone compounds are stronger.

Whether gingerols are converted into shogaols or zingerones, they have an incredible effect on the herb's flavor and medicinal properties. Shogaols result in the ginger exhibiting a more pungent flavor, while zingerones tend to be sweet. However, shogaols have a greater medicinal value due to the presence of alpha- and beta-unsaturated ketone moieties, which have both antioxidant and anti-inflammatory effects.

Ginger vitamins are also relevant when it comes to inflammation relief and management, mainly due to the high content of vitamin C (ascorbic acid) in this root. For those who prefer eating fresh, raw ginger, 100 grams of the root provide 5 mg of this powerful antioxidant, which helps repair and prevent the damage caused by free radicals. In that way, vitamin C not only contribute to slow the aging process, but also helps treating and preventing serious health conditions that are the consequence of chronic inflammation, such as arthritis and heart disease.

It should be noted that the vitamin C in ginger will break down as a result of heat and prolonged storage or exposure to light. Therefore, in order to reap both anti-inflammatory and antioxidant ginger effects, it is best to consume the fresh root. On the other hand, dried, powdered ginger has the most potent medicinal value due to its high shogaol levels. When taking the herb in this form, a daily dose of two to four grams is recommended.

Drinking ginger as a ginger tea, ginger water, ginger juice, or ginger extract has shown to be an effective remedy for soothing digestive ailments or nausea. It can even be applied topically, though it may cause some skin irritation. Ginger supplements may also be taken for treating nausea and inflammatory purposes.

Another great anti-inflammatory herb is turmeric. While the active anti-inflammatory effects of ginger are due to the inhibition of PH synthetase by gingerols, shogaols, and zingerones, turmeric's most significant active compounds are turmerone and curcumin. Turmerone inhibits the production of pro-inflammatory cytokines, while curcumin deactivates amyloid proteins, which have been linked to neurodegenerative diseases.

Though they work in different ways, both ginger and turmeric are very effective anti-inflammatory agents and can be used for different purposes.

(herbazest, 2019)

https://www.herbazest.com/herbs/ginger/ginger-for-inflammation

Promotes Proper Digestion

One of the most powerful ginger benefits is its ability to support digestive health and prevent problems like dyspepsia, a common condition of impaired digestion characterized by symptoms like pain, heartburn, fullness and discomfort. This study shows how Ginger speeds up the digestion process https://www.ncbi.nlm.nih.gov/pmc/articles/PMC3016669/ and this one shows consuming Ginger with your meal speeds up digestion too. https://www.ncbi.nlm.nih.gov/pubmed/18403946

(Dr. Jockers, 2019)

Ginger is one of my all-time favorite superfood herbs that I recommend to nearly every client I have ever worked with for its powerful ability to improve our digestive function and immune system. Superfoods such as ginger are foods and herbs that have a unique concentration of nutrients that synergize together to boost potential.

These foods are typically loaded with a combination of critical fatty acids, anti-oxidant phytonutrients and essential amino acids. Ginger is a classic example of this as it has compounds with health benefits that go far beyond what can be studied at this time.

Ginger is used throughout the world in countries such as China, Japan, India, Greece, Caribbean countries, England and the USA. It is made into teas, gingerale, beers, bread, snap cookies and biscuits. Almost every culture has historically used it for its powerful ability to enhance immunity, improve digestion and reduce inflammation.

This incredible superfood herb is 13th on the anti-oxidant list boasting an impressive ORAC score of 28,811. Ginger is composed of several volatile oils that give it it's characteristic flavor and odor; zingerone, shogaols, & gingerols. These oils are powerful anti-bacterial, anti-viral, anti-fungal, anti-parasitic agents (1). In addition, it inhibits cancer cell formation while firing up our body's own inborn ability to destroy the cancer cells formerly present.

Ginger has classically been used to improve the digestion process. Nine different substances have been found that stimulate serotonin receptors in the gut which provides benefits to the gastrointestinal system. This reduces gut related inflammation and enhances nutrient absorption.

Ginger is classified as a carminative (reducing intestinal gas) and an intestinal spasmolytic (soothes intestinal tract) while inducing gut motility. Ginger is known to reduce fever related nausea, motion sickness, and feelings of "morning sickness." Additionally, it helps aid in the production of bile, making it particularly helpful in digesting fats.

If you are dealing with digestive challenges, I highly encourage trying out ginger in your diet and health routine. Using some ginger tea on a daily basis is a great way to begin. We also have a fantastic de-inflaming ginger-ale recipe at the bottom of this article.

Ginger is also an important part of a de-inflaming, natural pain-relief program. One compound called 6-gingerol has been shown to significantly inhibit the production of a highly reactive nitrogen molecule, nitric oxide, that quickly forms a dangerous free radical peroxynitrite.

Additionally, ginger helps to protect the bodies stores of glutathione (the super anti-oxidant and free radical destroyer) (8, 9). Due to its effect on glutathione and nitric oxide, ginger has been shown to protect the brain and nervous system from degenerative stress (10).

Ginger is also very high in potassium which aids in electrical energy production and detoxification. It is a great source of manganese which protects the lining of the heart blood vessels and urinary tract. Ginger contains silicon which enhances skin, hair, teeth & nails. It helps assimilate calcium and reduces inflammation in the bone tissue aiding the development of strong bones and teeth.

Personally, ginger is something I recommend for a majority of my clients to use on a regular basis. This includes using ginger in teas and grating the fresh root on salads and meats and in green juices. Sometimes, I recommend supplementing with detox products that have this herb as it helps to aid in digestive function and liver detoxification.

Ginger helps stimulate digestive juices such as hydrochloric acid from the stomach and bile from the liver and gall bladder. This is why it is good to have ginger on or with your largest meals of the day. The Asian culture has used ginger in many of their dishes and you can even find pickled ginger with grocery store sushi packs.

I recommend grating fresh ginger on meat, salads and stews. You can also use dry, powdered forms if you are unable to access fresh ginger. It is quite pungent so use it mildly and it will provide you with excellent health benefits.

The Europeans developed gingerale many years ago and it was thought to be health tonic that would benefit a wide variety of ailments. That is until the 20th century when it became highly processed and full of sugar and artificial flavorings. Traditional gingerale was simply fermented ginger tea. The fermentation process activates ginger's full nutritional potential and it produces enzymes and probiotics for a powerful digestive health formula.

My de-inflaming gingerale uses coconut water which is rich in electrolytes and low in fructose. The sugar in the coconut water provides the nourishment for the good microbes to flourish. As they metabolize the sugar they produce B vitamins and organic acids that give the drink it's natural effervescence and characteristic flavor. You should be able to find a coconut water kefir starter called Inner Eco at your local health food store.

2 Tbsp of Coconut Water Kefir

1-2 cups of coconut water

2-4 oz of fresh ginger grated

Combine all ingredients and let sit and ferment for 24 hours to provide an amazing, probiotic enriched soda alternative.

Ginger has powerful anti-inflammatory and anti-microbial properties and is very effective in a blend of complementary supplements for a variety of health conditions. One of the key areas my team uses ginger for is to help the gut and reduce Candida and other opportunistic microbes such as H Pylori.

Ginger is one of my all-time favorite superfood herbs that I recommend to nearly every client I have ever worked with for its powerful ability to improve our digestive function and immune system. Superfoods such as ginger are foods and herbs that have a unique concentration of nutrients that synergize together to boost potential.

These foods are typically loaded with a combination of critical fatty acids, anti-oxidant phytonutrients and essential amino acids. Ginger is a classic example of this as it has compounds with health benefits that go far beyond what can be studied at this time.

Ginger is used throughout the world in countries such as China, Japan, India, Greece, Caribbean countries, England and the USA. It is made into teas, gingerale, beers, bread, snap cookies and biscuits. Almost every culture has historically used it for its powerful ability to enhance immunity, improve digestion and reduce inflammation.

This incredible superfood herb is 13th on the anti-oxidant list boasting an impressive ORAC score of 28,811. Ginger is composed of several volatile oils that give it it's characteristic flavor and odor; zingerone, shogaols, & gingerols. These oils are powerful anti-bacterial, anti-viral, anti-fungal, anti-parasitic agents (1). In addition, it inhibits cancer cell formation while firing up our body's own inborn ability to destroy the cancer cells formerly present.

Ginger has classically been used to improve the digestion process. Nine different substances have been found that stimulate serotonin receptors in the gut which provides benefits to the gastrointestinal system. This reduces gut related inflammation and enhances nutrient absorption. Ginger is classified as a carminative (reducing intestinal gas) and an intestinal spasmolytic (soothes intestinal tract) while inducing gut motility. Ginger is known to reduce fever related nausea, motion sickness, and feelings of "morning sickness." Additionally, it helps aid in the production of bile, making it particularly helpful in digesting fats.

If you are dealing with digestive challenges, I highly encourage trying out ginger in your diet and health routine. Using some ginger tea on a daily basis is a great way to begin. We also have a fantastic de-inflaming ginger-ale recipe at the bottom of this article.

Ginger has powerful anti-inflammatory and anti-microbial properties and is very effective in a blend of complementary supplements for a variety of health conditions. One of the key areas my team uses ginger for is to help the gut and reduce Candida and other opportunistic microbes such as H Pylori.

Our product Candida Elim features a bioavailable along with oregano, turmeric, olive leaf and caprylic acid. This is a fantastic product to support gut health and reshaping of the microbiome.

We also use ginger in combination with curcumin, boswelia, rosemary extract, systemic enzymes and bioflavonoids in our Inflam Defense. This combination of compounds is powerful for reducing inflammation in the body.

If you are dealing with chronic or acute pain conditions, degenerative joints or have elevated inflammatory markers on your lab testing than I would highly recommend the Inflam Defense product.

We also use ginger in combination with curcumin, boswelia, rosemary extract, systemic enzymes and bioflavonoids in our Inflam Defense. This combination of compounds is powerful for reducing inflammation in the body.

If you are dealing with chronic or acute pain conditions, degenerative joints or have elevated inflammatory markers on your lab testing than I would highly recommend the Inflam Defense product.

(Dr. Jockers, 2019) https://drjockers.com/10-ways-ginger-improves-digestion/

Sex and Increasing Testosterone Levels

Many talk about using Ginger as an aphrodisiac. I believe Ginger is an excellent tonic for men over the age of 50. It will increase your energy levels as well as your testosterone. This study agrees with this. https://www.ncbi.nlm.nih.gov/pubmed/30360442

Only a few natural testosterone boosters are supported by scientific studies. The herb with the most research behind it is called ashwagandha. One study tested the effects of this herb on infertile men and found a 17% increase in testosterone levels and a 167% increase in sperm count. In healthy men, ashwagandha increased levels by 15%. Another study found it lowered cortisol by around 25%, which may also aid testosterone.

Ginger extract may also boost your levels. It is a delicious herb that also provides various other health benefits. Most of the research on ginger has been done in animals. However, one study in infertile humans found that ginger can boost testosterone levels by 17% and increase levels of other key sex hormones. Other popular herbs that are supported by some studies in both animals and humans include horny goat weed, Mucuna pruriens, shilajit and tongkat ali. Yet it's important to note that most of the positive research has been conducted in mice or infertile humans with low testosterone levels. If you have healthy testosterone function and normal levels, it is unclear whether you will benefit much from these supplements.

Bottom Line: Several herbal supplements are a natural way to boost testosterone for those with infertility or low levels.

(reachmd, 2019) https://reachmd.com/news/8-proven-ways-to-increase-testosterone-levels-naturally/320/

I have been taking ginger powder in water for a few years and I agree with these findings. Ginger definitely increases testosterone, which makes you feel much younger and sexier. Ginger is truly magic how it can signifigantly reduce the effects of aging. I am also sure if you take herbs like ginger, astragalus and ashwagandah every day and follow the Blue Zone lifestyle you may feel young: no matter what the calendar says.

Eating Ginger

Ginger root can be eaten fresh or ground, juiced or infused into your favorite beverages. Ginger root pills are also available in tablet or capsule form to supply you with a quick and concentrated dose of antioxidants.

You can also use ginger to make a homemade cough syrup by boiling it in water with some honey or sugar. Ginger root is delicious in food and drinks. Ginger is used a lot in Asian stir fries and soups along with garlic and chili: a very healthy combination. Dr Keith Scott-Mumby has written a lot about how our bodies can tolerate a certain amount of abuse from junk food and a sedentary life tyle but there is a red line, once crossed, you quickly become ill because your body has lost its ability to fight disease. I agree with this: everything good thing you can do for your body counteracts every bad thing you do: it is so much better when the good far outweighs the bad. Taking Ginger every other day will help you on this quest.

Ginger root tea or ginger water is the perfect remedy for a queasy stomach, a bout of the flu or a long, stressful day. It's easy to prepare both of these beverages if you keep a steady supply of fresh and powdered ginger in your home.

Use a 2-inch knob of fresh ginger root and cut it into very thin slices. Add the ginger slices to hot water and boil for 10-30 minutes, depending on how strong you want it to be. Remove from the heat, strain and discard the ginger pieces and add in your choice of lemon, raw honey to enhance the flavor. Drink it hot as a tea or cool with ice.

Juicing ginger is pretty easy. Use the juice as a small shot or in your cooking. I often make ginger beer with grated fresh ginger, this is delicious.

You can store fresh ginger in a bag in your crisper drawer of your refrigerator for a couple of weeks: 3–4 weeks, or even longer with proper storage.

In moderation, ginger is generally safe and unlikely to cause any adverse side effects in most people. Common symptoms include stomach discomfort, heartburn and diarrhea.

If you experience any food allergy symptoms like hives, swelling or difficulty breathing, stop use immediately and talk to your doctor.

If taking ginger capsules, always start with a low dose and work your way up to assess your tolerance. Stick to the recommended dosage and decrease as needed if you have any negative symptoms.

Side effects

Heartburn, Skin irritation, swelling, and redness

Case Report
  Nosebleed, slow blood clotting: In a 76-year-old woman on long-term blood-thinning therapy who took ginger products. Clotting returned to normal after discontinuing ginger and with vitamin K administration.

Contraindications

Ginger supplements should not be used in the perioperative setting due to the potential risk for increased bleeding. This is in line with a general caution to avoid herbs that have antiplatelet and anticoagulation properties due to perioperative bleeding concerns, although a systematic review found inconclusive evidence. Likewise, ginger supplements should be avoided in patients with bleeding disorders.

Ginger supplements should be avoided during pregnancy or lactation due to lack of data on human fetal outcomes and concerns regarding embryo development in animal studies. The German Commission E also contraindicates ginger for morning sickness during pregnancy.

Individuals with gallstones should avoid ginger supplements due to potential cholagogic effects.

Herb drug interactions

Nonsteroidal anti-inflammatory drugs (NSAIDs): Ginger may increase bleeding tendency with concomitant use of drugs such as diclofenac or ibuprofen .

• Anticoagulants / Antiplatelets: Because ginger can inhibit thromboxane formation and platelet aggregation, concomitant use with anticoagulants may increase the risk of bleeding, although a systematic review determined that current evidence is inconclusive. Further study is warranted .

• Hypoglycemics / Insulin: Ginger may cause additive reductions in blood glucose.

• Tacrolimus: Pretreatment with ginger increases the plasma levels of tacrolimus.

• Cyclosporine: Concomitant use with ginger resulted in decreased blood concentrations of cyclosporine in vivo .

Do not take it if

You are taking warfarin or other blood thinners: Ginger supplements may increase the risk of bleeding.

You are taking NSAIDs, nonsteroidal anti-inflammatory drugs: Ginger supplements may increase bleeding tendency when used with these drugs.

You are taking insulin or medication to lower blood glucose: Ginger supplements may cause larger reductions in glucose levels.

You are taking tacrolimus: Ginger supplements increase the blood levels of this drug and may increase side effects.

You have a bleeding disorder: Ginger supplements may increase bleeding time.

You have gallstones: Ginger supplements may increase the flow of bile.

You are having surgery: Ginger supplements may increase bleeding risk.

You are pregnant or lactating: The effect of ginger supplements on the human gestational development are unknown.
(Dr. Axe, June 14 2018)

Turmeric

Tumeric is without a doubt the number one herb in the world. Thanks to heaps of research in the past five years thousands of people are successfully using turmeric to enhance their health in so many areas. The main ingredient of turmeric is curcumin. For general use, fresh and powdered turmeric with a pinch of black pepper will help improve many illnesses. For more serious and advanced conditions then it is important you purchase Curcumin (component of turmeric) with Bioperine. The research is in: turmeric is good for Alzheimer's, pain, inflammation, cancer, digestion, is antiviral and antibacterial. Used with coconut it is excellent brain food.

You can buy fresh turmeric at the market and cook curries with coconut oil, broccoli, and black pepper. It is easy to buy in powdered form from any herb shop. It is very cheap in Asia: $1 for 100 grams. Turmeric has a pretty good taste. I like to mix it with ginger powder and water and drink it before going to work. I have a friend who suffers from Gout and takes normal Gout medicine. I suggested turmeric and black pepper and after one month he has halved his medication. His blood pressure is back to normal too. There is so much scientific and anecdotal evidence about Turmeric on the internet I don't need to convince you to take it every other day: just let you know if you don't know yet, just how good it is.

Dr. Axe

https://draxe.com/turmeric-curcumin-benefits/
Dr. Axe, March 15, 2017
This is a complete extract of an article by Dr. Axe. Dr. Axe
is the first person you should follow for your health issues.
His articles are well researched and comprehensive. He
also has high-quality health products you can buy.

Turmeric (Curcuma longa), the main spice in the Indian
dish curry, is argued by many to be the most powerful
herb on the planet at fighting and potentially reversing
disease. Turmeric benefits are incredibly vast and very
thoroughly researched. Currently, there are over 12,500
peer-reviewed articles published proving turmeric
benefits, especially one of its renowned healing
compounds, curcumin. Curcumin is the active ingredient in
turmeric responsible for so many of its benefits. In fact,
turmeric is even good for dogs thanks to this active
ingredient.

This puts turmeric on top of the list as one of the most
frequently mentioned medicinal herbs in all of science. It
has a long history of use, particularly in Ayurvedic
medicine and other traditional forms of medicine. Here's
what you need to know about turmeric curcumin benefits
and more.

Turmeric comes from the Curcuma longa plant, which
grows in India and other Southeast Asian countries. It is a
member of the ginger family. The dried root of the
Curcuma longa plant is ground into the distinctive yellow
turmeric powder, giving it the name golden spice.

Why is turmeric good for you? There are several chemical compounds found in turmeric, known as curcuminoids. The active substance in turmeric is curcumin. Curcumin is what makes turmeric a "functional food," defined by the Mayo Clinic as "foods that have a potentially positive effect on health beyond basic nutrition." These turmeric nutrients and vitamins help provide turmeric powder health benefits.

Tumeric May Slow or Prevent Blood Clots

In both lab and animal studies, the use of turmeric curcumin greatly reduces instances of platelet aggregation and potentially reduces the risk of blood clots forming.

One combination lab and animal study conducted in 1986 even suggests curcumin may be a preferable treatment method for people "prone to vascular thrombosis and requiring antiarthritic therapy." However, this result still needs to be replicated in human trials.

Turmeric Reduces Depression Symptoms

Although few studies have been conducted on humans, dozens of research trials have proven that turmeric benefits include being especially effective in reducing depression symptoms in laboratory animals. These results seem to be connected to the way curcumin impacts neurotransmitter function through the brain-derived neurotrophic factor. The journal Phytotherapy Research published the results of an amazing, innovative study in 2014. The study took 60 volunteers diagnosed with major depressive disorder and split the group to determine how patients treated by turmeric curcumin fared against fluoxetine and a combination of the two. Curcumin was equally effective as fluoxetine in managing depression by the six-week mark.

Since that breakthrough trial, at least two other studies have observed the impact of turmeric's major compound, curcumin, in patients with depression. The first involved 56 individuals (male and female), and the second involved 108 male participants. Both used a placebo but did not compare curcumin to any antidepressant, and both studies found that curcumin effectively reduced depression symptoms more than placebo.

Turmeric Fights Inflammation

Arguably, the most powerful aspect of curcumin is its ability to control inflammation. The journal Oncogene published the results of a study that evaluated several anti-inflammatory compounds and found that curcumin is among the most effective anti-inflammatory compounds in the world.

Several animal trials have been completed investigating the relationship of curcumin and Alzheimer's disease. In mice, it seems that curcumin "reverses existing amyloid pathology and associated neurotoxicity," a key feature of the progression of this neurological disease related to chronic inflammation. This study shows turmeric curcumin may help with Alzheimer's symptoms.

Turmeric Boosts Skin Health

Turmeric benefits include anti-inflammatory and antioxidant properties that have proven effective in treating multiple skin conditions. Turmeric benefits for skin include increasing "glow and luster" of the skin, speeding up wound healing, calming the pores to decrease acne and acne scarring, and controlling psoriasis flares. One uncontrolled pilot study involving 814 participants even suggests that turmeric paste could cure 97 percent of scabies cases within three to 15 days.

"Try my Turmeric Face Mask for Glowing Skin. Just keep in mind that turmeric can stain the skin, and it may cause an allergic reaction. Do a patch test by applying a dime-size amount to your forearm. Then, wait for 24–48 hours to check for any reaction before applying turmeric to your face."

Turmeric May Outperform Common Arthritis Drug

Because curcumin is known for its powerful anti-inflammatory and pain-reducing characteristics, a study was conducted on 45 rheumatoid arthritis patients to compare the benefits of curcumin in turmeric to the arthritis drug diclofenac sodium (an NSAID), which put people at risk of developing leaky gut and heart disease. The study split these volunteers into three groups: curcumin treatment alone, diclofenac sodium alone and a combination of the two. The results of the trial were eye-opening: The curcumin group showed the highest percentage of improvement in overall [Disease Activity Score] scores and these scores were significantly better than the patients in the diclofenac sodium group. More importantly, curcumin treatment was found to be safe and did not relate with any adverse events. Our study provides the first evidence for the safety and superiority of curcumin treatment in patients with active RA, and highlights the need for future large-scale trials to validate these findings in patients with RA and other arthritic conditions. A review of available randomized, controlled trials confirmed that, of the eight studies available fitting the criteria, "these [randomized clinical trials] provide scientific evidence that supports the efficacy of turmeric extract (about 1000 mg/day of curcumin) in the treatment of arthritis."

Turmeric Could Treat or Prevent Certain Cancers

Of all the various topics scientists have tackled in regards to curcumin and disease reversal, cancer (of various types, including prostate cancer) is one of the most thoroughly researched topics. It may help with prostate cancer, pancreatic cancer and other forms of cancer. In the words of global authorities like Cancer Research UK: A number of laboratory studies on cancer cells have shown that curcumin does have anticancer effects. It seems to be able to kill cancer cells and prevent more from growing. It has the best effects on breast cancer, bowel cancer, stomach cancer and skin cancer cells. A July 2017 animal study by researchers at Baylor Scott & White Research Institute found that curcumin may even be able to break through chemo-resistance in pancreatic ductal adenocarcinoma (PDAC), an aggressive form of pancreatic cancer.

Turmeric May Help Manage Diabetes

In 2009, Biochemistry and Biophysical Research Communications published a lab study out of Auburn University that explored the potential of curcuminoids to lower glucose levels. The study discovered that curcumin in turmeric is literally 400 times more potent than metformin (a common diabetes drug) in activating the enzyme AMPK (AMP-activated protein kinase). One compound produced by fermentation of curcumin, tetrahydrocurcumin, activated AMPK up to 100,000 times more than metformin in certain cells. AMPK activation is considered by researchers to be a "therapeutic target" for type 2 diabetes, meaning that figuring out how to activate this enzyme has major potential for developing more effective treatments for reducing insulin resistance and reversing diabetes.

One of the most common complications of diabetes is damage to nerves known as diabetic neuropathy, which takes several forms and can cause serious symptoms throughout the body from muscle weakness to blindness. A study conducted on rats found that supplementing with curcumin significantly reduced diabetic peripheral neuropathic pain (typically localized to feet, legs, arms and hands). Diabetic neuropathy can also lead to kidney failure. A meta-analysis of randomized, controlled trials confirmed that, in animals, curcumin protects the kidneys of diabetic subjects from the damage of diabetic nephropathy.

Turmeric Combats Obesity

A study published in the journal Biofactors showed that curcumin may help reduce proliferation (growth) of fat cells, based on lab results. The researchers found that the anti-inflammatory properties in curcumin were effective at suppressing the inflammatory processes of obesity, therefore helping to reduce obesity and its "adverse health effects."

Turmeric Supports Management of Inflammatory Bowel Disease and Irritable Bowel Syndrome

An in-depth analysis of all the studies evaluating curcumin's ability to manage ulcerative colitis found that one very well-designed trial tested curcumin plus mesalazine (the typical NSAID prescribed for this condition) against placebo plus mesalazine. Patients taking only placebo and mesalazine were over four times more likely to experience a relapse or flare-up of ulcerative colitis during the six months of the study, suggesting that turmeric benefits may include helping to maintain remission of this chronic disease.

One small pilot study investigated the benefit of curcumin supplementation for patients with ulcerative colitis and patients with Crohn's disease. Although the sample size was very small, all of the ulcerative colitis patients and four out of five Crohn's patients had marked improvements over two months, suggesting the need for additional research. It shows promise for irritable bowel syndrome and other inflammatory bowel disease symptoms.

Turmeric May Regulate Cholesterol

A study published by Drugs in R&D found that curcumin was comparable to atorvastatin at reducing oxidative stress and inflammation in the treatment of high cholesterol in humans. This was a follow-up on prior animal research finding similar results. However, a 2014 meta-analysis concluded that curcumin had no effect overall on blood cholesterol (together or split into LDL vs. HDL) or on triglycerides. The study author noted that these results may be due to short study durations and poor bioavailability of the studied curcumin formulations.

Further research is needed, but there is evidence that turmeric curcumin may help manage cholesterol levels.

Turmeric Works as a Natural Pain Reliever

One of the more widely accepted properties of curcumin in scientific communities is its ability to manage pain. Breakthrough studies and reviews (some in animals, others in humans) have found that curcumin may be a beneficial natural painkiller for:

Wound healing and burn pain

Post-operative pain

Inflammation-induced arthritic pain

Neuropathic pain caused by constriction injury

Orofacial pain (pertaining to mouth, jaws and face, most commonly related to dental issues) Sciatic nerve pain from chronic constrictive injury (57)

Arthritis/joint pain

Turmeric Aids in Detoxification

An important benefit of turmeric is its ability to detoxify the body. Every day, you are likely exposed to environmental and dietary toxins known as xenobiotics. These chemical substances and not generally present in the human body and are often associated with increased amounts of inflammation and higher risk of cancer.
  It seems that consumption of turmeric and its active compound, curcumin, can help the liver efficiently detoxify the body and alleviate some of the effects of dangerous carcinogens. This process operates in tandem with the antioxidant and anti-inflammatory agents of turmeric.

What Is Turmeric Used For? How to Use Turmeric Curcumin in Your Diet

Turmeric Recipes

You may be wondering how to use turmeric root powder. One of my favorite recipes to incorporate turmeric benefits in your diet is turmeric tea, sometimes referred to as liquid gold or golden milk. The health benefits of turmeric tea are just as amazing as fresh turmeric root health benefits. Also, consuming turmeric eggs for breakfast and curried carrot soup is an excellent way to get more turmeric in your diet.

"I enjoy using coconut flakes, gluten-free flour and turmeric to bread chicken or sprinkle turmeric in my hamburger meat. I like to call that one a "Power Burger," and there are many more turmeric recipes you can use."

Turmeric Supplements

Although using turmeric frequently in your cooking is a great way to take advantage of the spice, turmeric only contains about 3 percent absorbable curcumin in the powdered form used in food. Along with adding turmeric into your diet, you may also consider taking it or curcumin in supplement form — some high-quality turmeric pills contain up to 95 percent curcuminoids.

There are a few things to consider when purchasing a good turmeric supplement. For one, try to find a turmeric supplement containing black pepper to get the maximum absorbability, as turmeric and black pepper work in tandem. Second, consider a fermented turmeric pill or capsule — the pre-digestion process of fermentation helps you to absorb it more effectively. Next, look for a turmeric supplement with other supporting ingredients like ashwagandha, milk thistle, dandelion and peppermint. Last, make sure that the product you get is made from organic turmeric if at all possible, with no GMOs. Note that turmeric dosage recommendations vary depending on a number of factors.

When is the best time of day to take turmeric supplements? Research varies, but it's believed that taking antioxidant supplements, such as turmeric curcumin, at bedtime may be most effective.

Turmeric Essential Oil

Turmeric is also available as an essential oil, which can be used alongside turmeric in food and supplement form. I personally prefer consuming a CO2-extracted form of turmeric essential oil. Quality is key here, particularly if you're going to use turmeric essential oil internally. Always dilute in water or other liquids. For example, you can put one drop in a smoothie in the morning.

Turmeric Side Effects and Caution

What are the side effects of turmeric? Turmeric might be allergic to some, as some people have reported allergic reactions to turmeric, especially after skin exposure. Typically this is experienced as a mild, itchy rash. In addition, high doses of turmeric have been observed to cause side effects of turmeric curcumin, including:

Nausea

Diarrhea

Increased risk of bleeding

Increased liver function tests

Hyperactive gallbladder contractions

Hypotension (lowered blood pressure)

Uterine contractions in pregnant women

Increased menstrual flow

If you experience these symptoms, stop using turmeric and get the medical advice of your doctor.

Final Thoughts on Turmeric Curcumin

Turmeric herb is one of the top nutrients in the world, whether we're talking turmeric powder, turmeric extract or turmeric pills. It has a long history of use, particularly in Ayurvedic medicine and other traditional forms of medicine.

What turmeric does for the body is amazing. Health-wise turmeric curcumin benefits range in everything from helping with blood clots and depression to combating inflammation, boosting skin health, regulating cholesterol and more.

I highly recommend using turmeric in recipes and perhaps even purchasing it in supplement form to take advantage of turmeric benefits. Make sure to add only organic turmeric to your food, and finding a high-quality turmeric supplement made from organic turmeric, coupled with black pepper and preferably prepared by fermentation.

Medical Disclaimer

their doctors or qualified health professionals regarding specific health questions. Neither Dr. Axe nor the publisher of this content takes responsibility for possible health consequences of any person or persons reading or following the information in this educational content. All viewers of this content, especially those taking prescription or over-the-counter medications, should consult their physicians before beginning any nutrition, supplement or lifestyle program.

https://draxe.com/turmeric-curcumin-benefits/
(Dr. Axe, March 15, 2017)

References

Turmeric

https://nccih.nih.gov/health/turmeric/ataglance.htm

Benefits of turmeric – Wellness Mama

https://wellnessmama.com/5297/turmeric-uses/

Turmeric – The spice of life – Dr. Mercola

https://www.acoi.org/sites/default/files/uploads/education/20 16-convention/Simon.pdf

Turmeric Life

https://www.turmericlife.com.au/

Memorial Sloan Kettering Cancer Center

https://www.mskcc.org/cancer-care/integrative-medicine/herbs/turmeric

NCBI

A review of its' effect on human health
https://www.ncbi.nlm.nih.gov/pmc/articles/PMC5664031/

Theraputic roles of curcumin
https://www.ncbi.nlm.nih.gov/pmc/articles/PMC3535097/

Turmeric the golden spice

https://www.ncbi.nlm.nih.gov/books/NBK92752/

Turmeric for arthritis

https://www.ncbi.nlm.nih.gov/pmc/articles/PMC5003001/

Turmeric uses in a broad range of treatments
https://www.ncbi.nlm.nih.gov/pmc/articles/PMC5852989/

Conclusion

Pharmaceuticals, supplements and herbal products are quite often expensive. I think you should build your health routine on all the cheap, organic and fresh herbs you can buy at your local market or grow your self. Most of us live our lives feeling like we don't have enough money and there is no greater culprit for this than pharmaceutical companies with their pretty packaging and gigantic markups.

If one reason you don't take many herbs is because they are expensive then keep reading. Food is our medicine: period. Herbs are part of our food: much more so in Asia than in Western countries. So if herbs are part of our food then we need to buy herbs like food and eat them like food. Countries like India have such an amazing array of herbs and spices they use to cook their food. When they take their herbs for their health they are not ordering them from Amazon or buying them off the shelf in a pharmacy, they are just eating them like food from their garden and local market. This knowledge is enough to change your life forever. Learn about food is our medicine every day. Broccoli is the best example by far. This yummy green vegetable is now being used by pharmaceutical companies to make products to sell you at very high prices. Why are they doing this? Because sulfurane in broccoli is an incredible cancer cure and preventative. This makes broccoli a herb, medicine, and food. You need to buy organic or grow your own to get the full benefits of food being your medicine. If it is full of Monsanto's Roundup then it will kill you not save you.

Ginger and Turmeric are very easy to grow; along with garlic, chilies and red onions. There is a huge list of herbs you can grow that will transform your life. There is a conflict of interest in chemical companies like Monsanto poisoning you and then their sister company selling you $400,000 worth of chemotherapy drugs to cure you of what the roundup did: give you cancer.

If you have no room to grow these herbs and don't know where to buy them then there are lots of herb companies on the internet that you can use like Mountain Rose Herbs https://www.mountainroseherbs.com/products/ginger-root-powder/profile

It's up to you break free of a system based around profits and not people. The profit motive of so many people is destroying our world. There is no future for any of us if the rich only want to get richer and more powerful and continue to widen the gap between normal people than them. One way to stop this is to stop buying their 'stuff' and make your own. If you think you are going to the supermarket to buy food because it's convenient: you are wrong. You are going because they are changing the world around you, making you a consumer, encouraging you to depend on "mass produced food" so they can make money, money,x, and more money: there is little profit in one organic carrot: but lots of nutrition.

Thank you so much for buying this book and listening to these words. Ginger and turmeric have really changed my life so I hope they can change yours too.

Roditch.